Intermittent Fasting: Ultimate Guide to Health with Intermittent Fasting

Heal Mind, Body, and Soul with Intermittent Fasting

Dr. Michelle Danville

Disclaimer:

© 2017 – TWK - Publishing. All Rights Reserved.

No part of this publication may be reproduced, stored or transmitted in any form or by any means – electronic, mechanical, scanning, photocopying, recording or otherwise, without prior written permission from the author.

This publication is provided for informational and educational purposes only and cannot be used as a substitute for expert medical advice. The information contained herein does not take into account an individual reader's health or medical history.

Hence, it's important to consult with a health care professional before starting any regimen mentioned herein. Though all possible efforts have been made in the preparation of this eBook, the author makes no warranties as to the accuracy or completeness of its contents.

The readers understand that they can follow the information, guidelines and ideas mentioned in this eBook at their own risk. All trademarks mentioned are the property of their respective owners.

Table of Contents

Introduction

I want to thank you and congratulate you for downloading *Intermittent Fasting: Ultimate Guide to Health with Intermittent Fasting.*

I have probably tried more than a dozen of diet plans that can help me lose weight and none gave me the results I wanted to see. I decided to go on a diet when my health began to deteriorate. I could no longer fit in my favorite dress and my self-confidence plunged.

I get tired easily and could not focus well on my work. I was restless and my spirit seemed to have lost its usual vigor. I gave up the diet plans, which did not help at all, and then a friend introduced me to intermittent fasting.

I was skeptical and did not want to bother with it but I still tried it after my friend told me about the wonderful benefits that she gained. I found it hard to adjust to the program because intermittent fasting is way different from the diet programs that I've tried. Soon, I noticed my body becoming light and I was able to move faster than before. I lose weight and gained muscle mass. I was able to gain back my self-esteem and confidence. My health has greatly improved.

Today, I can wear my favorite dress again. I can walk the streets with confidence while wearing jeans and sleeveless top. I feel light and I can move with ease.

This book provides a thorough guide to intermittent fasting to help you make the program work for you too. The book contains:

- A brief explanation about what intermittent fasting is.

- Types of intermittent fasting.

- Foods and meal preparations that can help you achieve the results that you want to see.

- Ways to suppress the urges to eat.

- Explanation regarding autophagy.

- How to do a proper workout with intermittent fasting.

- Other important information that you would like to know and help you reach your goal in a matter of time.

If you have tried so many diet plans, you too may get overwhelmed by the difference – at first. It would be a lot easier as time goes by. Also, keep in mind to set a realistic goal to avoid frustrations.

Intermittent fasting can do wonders for you. It is still advisable to seek your doctor's opinion first before you try any diet program.

Thanks again for purchasing this book, I hope you enjoy it!

Chapter 1

What is Intermittent Fasting?

Intermittent fasting is an eating pattern that follows a cycle of eating and fasting. It does not restrict the type of foods that you eat, although eating more organic vegetables and fruits can help a lot. It is far from the usual diet programs that require food planning, including what you must eat or not eat. It is more focused on when you should eat your meal and not what kinds of food you need to eat.

Your eating pattern is your utmost concern when you follow intermittent fasting. Here is a list of typical intermittent fasting schedules:

- Fasting for 12 hours on daily basis.

- Fasting for 16 hours on daily basis.

- Fasting for 20 hours, one or two times each week.

- Fasting for 24 hours, one or two times each week.

Here is a sample table for 16-hour fasting:

	Sunday	Monday	Tuesday	Wednesday	Thursday	Friday	Saturday
Midnight	Fasting	Fasting	Fasting	Fasting	Fasting	Fasting	Fasting
4:00 AM	Fasting	Fasting	Fasting	Fasting	Fasting	Fasting	Fasting
8:00 AM	Fasting	Fasting	Fasting	Fasting	Fasting	Fasting	Fasting
12:00 PM	First meal at 12pm	First meal at 12pm	First meal at 12pm	First meal at 12pm	First meal at 12pm	First meal at 12pm	First meal at 12pm
4:00 PM	Last meal around 8pm	Last meal around 8pm	Last meal around 8pm	Last meal around 8pm	Last meal around 8pm	Last meal around 8pm	Last meal around 8pm
8:00 PM	Fasting	Fasting	Fasting	Fasting	Fasting	Fasting	Fasting
Midnight	Fasting	Fasting	Fasting	Fasting	Fasting	Fasting	Fasting

You can adjust the table if you want to have your first meal at 8:00 a.m. and your last meal for the day at 4:00 p.m. You can also follow any of these schedules (just replace the time on the given table):

- If at 7:00 a.m. you have your first meal, your last meal should be around 3:00 p.m. and you then begin your 16 hours of fasting.

- If at 11:00 a.m. you have your first meal, your last meal should be around 7:00 p.m. and then your 16 hours of fasting should commence.

- If at 2:00 p.m. you have your first meal, your last meal should be around 10:00 p.m.

and after that you must not eat anything for the next 16 hours.

- If at 6:00 p.m. you have your first meal, your last meal should be around 2:00 a.m. and you need to fast for 16 hours after you finished your food.

You are still considered fasting when you are already sleeping. The important thing to remember is that you should not eat anything anymore during your fasting hours. In a day, you need to miss at least one meal.

One of the Most Popular Fitness Trends

Currently, intermittent fasting is one of the most popular health and fitness trends in the world. There are many studies that show it can help you lose weight, fight off disease, enhance metabolic health, and may even make it possible for you to live longer.

The different intermittent fasting methods only have eating periods and fasting periods in their schedule. The truth is all people "fast" each day even if they don't practice intermittent fasting. They fast while they sleep, work an important task, or anything that made them unable to eat anything. Intermittent fasting is a practice that extends the time that you don't get to eat anything for a bit longer than normal.

You can extend it by skipping at least one meal per day. Most people believe that breakfast is the most important meal of the day and it is foolish to skip it. When you have decided to do intermittent fasting, you can always regard your first meal of the day as your breakfast.

No matter what time you have decided to take it. Think that in some other parts of the world, people are taking their breakfast at the same moment you are taking yours. You may be taking your breakfast at noon but in some other places it's morning.

When you have decided to do intermittent fasting, you may experience adjustment phase. There are lots of people who say that they feel better and more energetic during a fast. You may feel extremely hungry during the first few days of fasting, but your body will be able to adapt to your new eating habits as time goes by. You won't even mind skipping one or two meals a day because you won't feel hunger pains.

You are not allowed to eat anything during fasting periods, but you can drink water. You are also allowed to drink tea, coffee, homemade fruit infused water, coconut water, and other drinks that don't contain calories. If you find it difficult to swallow tasteless water all the time, prepare fruit infused water.

Just add some slices of fruit and/or herb in your water, stir or mash for a bit, and let it stand at room temperature before you refrigerate it. You can prepare it beforehand so you will have a refreshing drink later. Commercially produced fruit infused water contains loads of sugar, which is not good for your health. It is also advisable to stay away from sports drinks.

There are some intermittent fasting methods that allow you to eat small amounts of foods that have low calories during your fasting period. You can also take some supplements during fasting period and remember that they should not contain any calorie.

Why there's a Need to Fast

People have been fasting for centuries and no one could really tell the exact time when it all began. Various religions, including Buddhism, Christianity, and Islam require their members to practice fasting. Sometimes, the absence of food or unavailability of source compels someone to fast.

Humans as well as animals, instinctively fast whenever they feel unwell. There is nothing strange about fasting. Our bodies can handle long periods of not eating anything. In fact, Mahatma Gandhi successfully endured 21 days of not consuming any food. However, it is different with water. You can only make it through 100 hours without drinking any liquid under average temperature. Your body gets dehydrated fast under extreme heat.

When you fast, your blood sugar and insulin levels will naturally go down. There's also a drastic rise in growth hormone.

Many people turn to intermittent fasting to lose weight. It is a simple and effective way to burn fat and to restrict calories. Others take advantage of metabolic health benefits that intermittent fasting provides.

Some research suggests that intermittent fasting can prolong your life as it helps protect your body against diseases, which include Alzheimer's, cancer, type 2 diabetes, and heart disease.

On the practical sense, you can actually save some money when you practice intermittent fasting. You only need to worry about your two meals per day instead of three or four. You also save time when you don't need to prepare and clean as much as before whenever you take your meal. Best of all, you will feel light, fit, and healthy. Intermittent fasting also brings amazing benefits to your spirit and mind.

How does it Work?

To understand how intermittent fasting works, you need to know first what actually happens during an eating period and a fasting period.

During eating period, your body digests and absorbs food. Eating period usually lasts up to 8 hours (depending on the type of intermittent fasting that you would like to follow). When you are eating, your insulin level becomes high and it prevents your body from burning fat. Insulin lets your body use glucose as fuel. Once eating period ends, your body goes through post-absorptive state (a fancy name or term that means your body is not processing food).

When your eating period ends, your fasting period begins. During fasting period, it is very convenient for your body to burn fat because of your low insulin level. Understand that your insulin level won't automatically go down after you have your last meal for the day. It may take some time (usually after three to five hours after eating your last meal) before your body begins to burn fat. Your body is in fat burning state during fasting.

Who are not allowed to fast?

Although fasting is something beneficial, not all people can be allowed to do it. You should not fast if you are any of the following:

1. Pregnant

A pregnant woman must provide added nutrients that her child needs and should not skimp on her diet. Although, she should still watch what she eats or she may experience difficult delivery when her child becomes too big. It is not advisable to practice intermittent fasting during pregnancy and it is wise to eat only nutritious foods that won't make the unborn child too big.

2. Breastfeeding

A child needs all the nutrients that he can get from milk provided by his mother. If you are currently nursing, it is best to think about ways to give all the nutrients that your child needs by eating properly. Forget about fasting and concentrate on your child's welfare first.

3. Underweight

If your BMI (body mass index) is less than 18.5, fasting may only bring detrimental effects to your health. Intermittent fasting can make you lose weight even if you don't intend to bring your weight down. If you are underweight, you need to eat more to reach your ideal weight. Losing more than your already unacceptable weight will only damage your health.

4. Under 18 years old

Children under 18 years old are still in their growing years and need extra nutrients to develop properly. Fasting can hinder a child's proper development. There are cases where doctors recommend fasting, but it is supervised or closely monitored. Someone who is below 18 years old should not even try fasting out of curiosity. Fasting may greatly affect a child's growing years.

People with high uric acid or gout, diabetes mellitus (type 1 or type 2), and those with prescription medication should not fast on their own. They can fast but they are not allowed to fast without a doctor's supervision. Individuals with eating disorder history should not try intermittent fasting. It is also best for women who are trying to conceive to drop any plan of practicing intermittent fasting or taking any diet program without their doctor's advice or supervision.

Important Tips to Remember

When you have just started your intermittent fasting, you may feel like you won't be able to make it through the fasting period because of hunger. Don't worry because most people who decided to follow intermittent fasting went through the same ordeal.

Here are some of the things that can help you curb your hunger:

1. Drink water, tea, or coffee to ease your hunger.

2. Keep yourself busy to keep your mind occupied and not to think about food.

3. Your hunger will eventually subside, so make sure not to give in.

4. You have just started, so give it a try for one month and don't give up easily.

5. It is best not to tell anybody who doesn't support your desire to practice intermittent fasting. Their negative attitude might affect your enthusiasm.

6. Remember not to binge after your fasting period ends.

Intermittent fasting can bring lots of benefits. If you are not allowed to engage in fasting, it is wise not to push it.

Chapter 2

History of Fasting and Benefits that it Brings

All throughout human history, people used fasting to recover from illnesses. Most written records mentioned fasting being used by people of different regions, race, gender, and religion. All suggests that fasting has shown effectiveness since long ago.

Fasting was used by priests, philosophers, and doctors. In ancient India and Egypt as well as Greece, dosed starvation (equivalent to fasting) was used for curative and preventive purposes. It was also used to strengthen the spirit.

According to Greek Historians

Greek Historian Herodotus (484 to 425 years BC) once said that among men, Egyptians are considered the healthiest. For three days in each month, they vomit to purify their body. They always believed that an individual could get ill through food.

Greek Philosopher and Mathematician Pythagoras (580 to 500 years BC) starved systematically for 40 days because he believed that such act would let him enhance his creativity and mental perception. When demanded a 40-day fast, he consumed nothing but water. He and his followers also ate strict vegetarian diet.

Greek Philosopher Plato (427 to 347 years BC), who is also Socrates' disciple, categorized medicine under "true" (provides health) or "false" (gives nothing but phantom health). Treatments by diet and fasting, sun, and air were all included under category "true".

Great Physician Hippocrates (460 to 357 years BC) once said that if you richly fed a patient, his disease would be fed as well. You need to keep in mind that any excess is considered bad.

Spiritual History of Fasting

The most widely read book in the history of man, The Holy Bible, has documented how fasting was performed during that time. Some fasts that were mentioned in the Bible were complete abstinence from water and food. The Bible has examples of a wide array of motivating factors for people to fast, such as to show repentance or grief.

Fasting for Forty Days

The earliest recorded fasting in the Bible happened during Moses' time. When God told him to go to Mount Sinai to receive the tablets that contain the Ten Commandments, he neither ate nor drank water. God miraculously made Moses abstain from eating and drinking water without making him ill. During Biblical times, God never failed to provide sustenance to His people whenever necessary. They only need to remain loyal and obey the set of rules every day. Those who acted against the commandments suffered great loss.

For the Forgiveness of Sin

The Holy Bible has narrated countless stories or accounts about people fasting to show their remorse and repentance. When you visit 1 Samuel 7:2, you will see that Samuel called a corporate fast when the people of Israel defied the law regarding idolatry. After they got rid of all idols in the land, people went to Mizpeh with Samuel. They fasted on that same day as they uttered their cry for forgiveness and openly admitted that they have sinned against the Lord.

People of Israel fasted whenever an event, which they know was not pleasing to God, happened. They fast to show their utmost sorrow for committing something unpleasant in the eyes of God and convey their deep repentance.

Modern Christians, especially those who are considered devotees, still do the same practice. For them, fasting can somehow make them feel that they have a better chance for the forgiveness of sins that they have committed. Although it is impossible to predict their chances of being forgiven, fasting can somehow provide comfort and ease to their mind, body, and soul.

Day of Atonement

God even told the people to fast on the appointed Day of Atonement. He required repentance and soul-searching while atonement was being carried out. God also declared the tenth day of the seventh month to be the Day of Atonement.

Fasting and Prayer

The Bible presents various paradigms of fasting combined with fervent prayer. In 1 Samuel 1:7 to 8, Hannah fasted and earnestly prayed to God to give her a child. In 2 Samuel 12:16, it depicted how David fasted and solemnly prayed for his infant son's health restoration. Even the good King Darius fasted and prayed for Daniel's safety while in a lion's den, and the full account can be found in the Book of Daniel.

There are other incidents that people from Biblical times combined fasting and prayer whenever they ask something from God to show their utmost sincerity.

Jesus on Fasting

Even Jesus left commandments and instructions regarding fasting to his disciples. He was expecting His followers to fast.

Jesus taught His followers to do the act without any aim of gaining some praise for their act or for any selfish reasons. To fast openly for others to know can be considered as something without value. Someone should not yearn to get praised for being a spiritual person. Jesus would remind His followers to fast in secret to get their reward from God. Right after teaching the Lord's Prayer to His disciples, Jesus talked about fasting.

The prayer is a perfect example of how one should submit peacefully to the will of God and to show the believer's acceptance of God's sovereignty. The pure humility that emanates from deep within is needed to conduct a meaningful fasting.

If you follow the accounts in the Bible regarding the life of Jesus and His teachings, you will learn that fasting was something they often do for a lot of different reasons. Fasting helped them achieved their goals and carried out their missions with success.

Fasting in the Modern World

Fasting still plays a significant role in the modern time. From the ancient time to the present, mankind relies on fasting for good health and spiritual reasons.

Friedrich Hoffman (1660 to 1742) is a physician who widely used limotherapy, which is a short voluntary abstinence from food in alternative medicine. It can be used to alleviate different diseases. Dr. Hoffmann's first rule was that each patient should not eat anything while under his prescribed treatment.

Friedrich Hufeland (1762 to 1836), founder of rational hygiene and author of "The Macrobiotic and the Art of Prolonging Human Life", also believed that patients should abstain from eating. He reasoned that patients will only find it difficult to digest food and will only contribute to the worsening of the ailment.

In 1877, an American doctor named Edward Dewey began using long-term fasting in an attempt to gain curative effects. He explained that for diseases that lead to loss of appetite and occurrence of coated tongue, a patient should avoid eating until his appetite comes back and his tongue becomes clear. Dr. Dewey was a supporter of prolonged fasting during his time.

Dr. Henry Tanner (1831 to 1919) was an American doctor just like Dr. Dewey who believed that fasting will bring curative benefits to his patients. He even declared that intermittent abstinence from food can be considered an elixir in maintaining youth.

Other doctors, including Alexander Haig, Von Noorden, Maximillan Oskar Bircher-Benner, recognized limotherapy as a method that can be considered as a natural therapy. Other countries also recognized the beneficial contributions of fasting in healing patients from their illnesses.

Important Benefits of Fasting

Fasting can provide lots of benefits, including the following:

- Weight loss

- Enhanced senses

- Anti-aging effects

- Promotes better relaxation

- Clearer mind

- Improved mood and attitude

- Better immune system

- Fairer skin

- Mental and emotional clarity

- Energy boost

- Spiritual awareness

- Rest for the digestive system

- Rejuvenation

Fasting was not always well received by the public and health authorities. In fact, there were times when doctors who treated their patients using fasting as the method of treatment were often criticized. Despite opposition from pharmaceutical companies and other health professionals, fasting did not leave the limelight and continues to evolve.

Chapter 3

Types of Intermittent Fasting

There are different types of intermittent fasting, and all you need to do is choose the one that fits in with your schedule, preference, and tolerance. There are **evidences and studies** that can prove how intermittent fasting can help you lose weight and even lower your risk of acquiring chronic diseases.

12-Hour Fast

This type of intermittent fasting is recommended for newbies. You can change your schedule once you got the hang of it. As the name suggests, you have a fasting of 12 hours and an eating period of the same length of time. You can follow this table:

Intermittent Fasting

	Sunday	Monday	Tuesday	Wednesday	Thursday	Friday	Saturday
Midnight	Fasting	Fasting	Fasting	Fasting	Fasting	Fasting	Fasting
4:00 AM	Fasting	Fasting	Fasting	Fasting	Fasting	Fasting	Fasting
8:00 AM	Breakfast at 8am	Breakfast at 8am	Breakfast at 8am	Breakfast at 8am	Breakfast at 8am	Breakfast at 8am	Breakfast at 8am
12:00 PM	Lunch at 12pm	Lunch at 12pm	Lunch at 12pm	Lunch at 12pm	Lunch at 12pm	Lunch at 12pm	Lunch at 12pm
4:00 PM	Dinner around 8pm	Dinner around 8pm	Dinner around 8pm	Dinner around 8pm	Dinner around 8pm	Dinner around 8pm	Dinner around 8pm
8:00 PM	Fasting	Fasting	Fasting	Fasting	Fasting	Fasting	Fasting
Midnight	Fasting	Fasting	Fasting	Fasting	Fasting	Fasting	Fasting

If you usually sleep for 8 hours, you only need to think of things to do to curb your hunger for the remaining 4 hours of fasting when you are awake. Fasting for 12 hours may seem difficult but when you think about it, you are mostly fast asleep within the 12-hour time frame allotted for fasting.

With this type of intermittent fasting, you can still eat your three meals (perhaps some snacks too). When fasting periods begins, you must absolutely prevent yourself from eating anything. You are still allowed to drink water and other liquids that have no sugar. It is highly recommended to have low-calorie foods during your eating period.

The 8-Hour Window or 16/8 Method

This type of intermittent fasting is also called Leangains protocol, which fitness expert Martin Berkhan popularized. For a beginner, this method may be too much to handle that's why I suggested the 12-hour fast first. If you think you need more than 12 hours of fasting and can handle it, this method might just be the one you need.

It involves fasting for 14 to 16 hours every day, and eating period is restricted to 8 to 10 hours. This means skipping breakfast and not eating anything after dinner. A sample table was already given in Chapter 1.

Many people who often skip breakfast finds this method suitable, but those who are used to eating breakfast immediately upon waking up may eventually get used to it after a few days or weeks. When you drink liquids during the fast, choose water, tea, and other beverages that have no calories.

It is recommended to eat foods that contain more calories and carbs during training days and more fats on your rest days. As a constant reminder, eat only nutritious foods and stay away from junk foods.

It may take a long time before you see any positive change in your health and fitness if you keep consuming junk foods during eating period. It is also impossible to achieve your goal if you keep eating unhealthy foods.

There are also **studies** that can prove this type of intermittent fasting can help hinder occurrence of diabetes, liver disease, and obesity.

20:4 Method

This requires daily fasting for 20 hours. This type of intermittent fasting only requires 4 hours of eating. When you choose to do this, you can eat anytime and anything (make sure it's nutritious, though) within the 4-hour time frame. After 4 hours, you begin fasting for the next 20 hours. You can also do this type of fasting on a daily basis or anywhere between once and thrice a week.

For example, let us say that you have decided to eat your meals between 12:00 p.m. and 4:00 p.m. This means you need to skip breakfast, eat your lunch at 12:00 p.m., and should have eaten your supper by 4:00 p.m. After consuming your last meal for the day, you begin your fasting period.

The 5:2 Plan

This type of intermittent fasting involves eating normal healthy meals for five days, and then restricting your caloric intake to only 500 (for women) to 600 (for men) calories for the next two days. This is also known as Fast Diet, which Dr. Michael Mosley popularized.

It may be quite difficult to follow at first or you may also choose to follow other type of intermittent fasting that is more suitable for you. Insisting on a 5:2 method won't be a wise decision if you can't even do it properly.

You can start with less than 100 calories breakfast, less than 200 calories lunch, and 200 to 400 calories dinner. Your meal should consist of lots of vegetables, protein, and good fats. Drink plenty of liquids to help curb your hunger. You still need to keep away from beverages that contain sugar.

24-Hour Fast

This involves fasting for a period of one day. You only need to eat one meal in a day and then you begin fasting. Let us say you have decided to fast after having your lunch. Your next meal will be lunch of the following day. You skip two meals on the day you start fasting and skip breakfast of the following day. You only need to do this type of fasting once or twice a week. There are others who can do it three times a week.

You can even start doing it once a week and gradually work your way to doing it three times in a week. Don't force your body too much. It is also important to know your limitations.

You may follow a schedule similar to the table below:

	Sunday	Monday	Tuesday	Wednesday	Thursday	Friday	Saturday
Midnight – 4:00 AM	Sleeping	Sleeping	Fasting	Sleeping	Sleeping	Sleeping	Sleeping
4:00 AM – 8:00 AM	Sleeping	Sleeping	Fasting	Sleeping	Sleeping	Sleeping	Sleeping
8:00 AM – 12:00 PM	Breakfast at 8am	Fasting	Fasting	Breakfast at 8am	Breakfast at 8am	Breakfast at 8am	Breakfast at 8am
12:00 PM – 4:00 PM	Lunch at 12pm	Lunch at 12pm	Lunch at 12pm	Lunch at 12pm	Lunch at 12pm	Lunch at 12pm	Lunch at 12pm
4:00 PM – 8:00 PM	Dinner at 8pm	Fasting	Dinner at 8pm	Dinner at 8pm	Dinner at 8pm	Dinner at 8pm	Dinner at 8pm
8:00 PM – Midnight	Resting	Fasting	Resting	Resting	Resting	Resting	Resting
Midnight	Sleeping	Fasting	Sleeping	Sleeping	Sleeping	Sleeping	Sleeping

Take note that on days that you don't fast, you can also eat snacks whenever you take a rest. I changed the labels to emphasize your real fasting period. The same goes with all sample tables with similar labels.

36-Hour Fast

This method involves fasting for a whole day and a half. For example (see table below), you eat your dinner at 8:00 p.m. on day 1, your fasting period begins after finishing your meal. On day 2, you will not eat anything and just fast for a whole day. You can drink water and beverages that contain no sugar and/or calories.

On day 3, you eat breakfast at 8:00 a.m. and follow your normal schedule. When you count the number of fasting hours, you will get 36. This method or type of intermittent fasting can provide a more powerful weight loss benefit.

	Day 1	Day 2	Day 3	Day 4	Day 5	Day 6	Day 7
Midnight – 4:00 AM	Sleeping	Fasting	Fasting	Sleeping	Sleeping	Sleeping	Sleeping
4:00 AM – 8:00 AM	Sleeping	Fasting	Fasting	Sleeping	Sleeping	Sleeping	Sleeping
8:00 AM – 12:00 PM	Working	Fasting	Breakfast at 8am	Breakfast at 8am	Breakfast at 8am	Breakfast at 8am	Breakfast at 8am
12:00 PM – 4:00 PM	Working	Fasting	Lunch at 12pm	Lunch at 12pm	Lunch at 12pm	Lunch at 12pm	Lunch at 12pm
4:00 PM – 8:00 PM	Dinner at about 8pm	Fasting	Dinner at about 8pm	Dinner at about 8pm	Dinner at about 8pm	Dinner at about 8pm	Dinner at about 8pm
8:00 PM – Midnight	Fasting	Fasting	Resting	Resting	Resting	Resting	Resting
Midnight	Fasting	Fasting	Sleeping	Sleeping	Sleeping	Sleeping	Sleeping

Alternate-Day Fasting

This method requires fasting every other day. There are actually different versions of this type of intermittent fasting. There's a version that incorporates the 5:2 method's diet plan of consuming only 500 to 600 calories during fasting period.

There's also a version wherein an individual should fast for a whole day and to do it alternately within a week. Beginners must absolutely avoid this version of alternate-day fasting.

The Warrior Diet

Ori Hofmekler popularized this method, wherein you fast during daytime and have a feast at night. The suggested food choices for this diet are similar to that of Paleo diet. You must eat only whole, unprocessed, and organic food – anything that can be harvested naturally and without any chemical. Your meat should be grass-fed and you must stay away from fruits and vegetables that have been sprayed with chemicals.

Spontaneous Meal Skipping

This type of intermittent fasting does not require you to follow a specific schedule. You simply skip meals from time to time

when you don't feel like eating or not hungry. You may choose to skip breakfast, and then eat nutritious lunch and dinner. This method is also ideal if you are someone
who frequently travels. Whenever you can't find anything to eat, you can always do a short fast. It is important to always consume healthy foods whenever you eat. Eliminate junk foods from your diet.

Extended Fasting

This type of intermittent fasting usually takes more than 48 hours of fasting period. Experts recommend taking multivitamins to prevent micronutrients deficiency. Fasting for 7 to 14 days is possible (remember Gandhi). However, it is not advisable to go more than 14 days of fasting.

Choose the system which you think will work for you. It is foolish to choose long hours of fasting in your first try. It is also advisable to start eating healthy foods now
and eliminate those that contain high amounts of sugar and chemicals.

Chapter 4

Eating the Right Foods and Breaking the Fast

You are allowed to eat anything you want when you have decided to practice intermittent fasting. However, it still helps a lot if you carefully plan your meal. Also, planning which foods can satisfy your hunger longer will make fasting easier to do. Eating fiber-rich foods can make you feel full longer than consuming just about anything that comes to mind. Proper planning is important if you want to make intermittent fasting works for you.

Eating the Right Foods

It is also important to choose the type of intermittent fasting that won't get in the way of your usual activities. Once you have chosen the most suitable one, you also need to plan the foods you eat that works well with the type of intermittent fasting that you want to practice.

On non-fast days, you can eat whatever you want but it is recommended to stick to healthy foods if you want to have a fit and healthy body in a matter of time. As a reminder you must:

- Choose organic, fresh produce.

- Avoid commercial beverages or drinks that contain too much sugar.

- Opt for grass-fed meat.

- Eliminate junk foods.

- Drink plenty of liquids.

- Exercise regularly.

- Never miss a routine check-up.

- Avoid excessive drinking, smoking, and illegal substance.

- Take vitamins and supplements as needed.

Before we go to the healthy meal plans for your non-fast days, checkout the good sources of quality carbohydrates, protein, and fats.

List of Quality Food Sources

As much as possible, you need to use foods that are regarded as high quality sources of your needed nutrients when drafting an effective meal plan.

Quality Carbohydrates

Carbohydrates of high quality can help your body maintain ideal levels of blood sugar and insulin as well as provide antioxidants.

The table below has a list of quality carbohydrates that you can include in your daily meals:

Class	Food
Vegetables	Yellow squash
	String beans
	Spinach
	Red pepper
	Onion
	Kale
	Eggplant
	Cucumber

	Celery
	Cauliflower
	Cabbage
	Brussels sprouts
	Romaine lettuce
	Broccoli
Fruits	Tomato
	Strawberries
	Red grapes
	Plum
	Pink Grapefruit
	Pear
	Kiwi
	Green grapes
	Blueberries
	Orange
	Blackberries

Quality Protein

Protein can help you build muscle mass and gives you power to get up and go. It can also help support cognitive function and mood. Research also suggests that many people need more high-quality protein as they age.

Below is a list of protein that you can include in your diet:

Class	Food
Top Protein Source	Turkey breast, deli
	Turkey breast
	Tuna steak
	Soybean hamburger crumbles
	Snapper
	Sea bass
	Salmon
	Mackerel
	Lobster
	Haddock
	Cod
Second Best Source of Protein	Tuna, canned in water
	Trout
	Soy imitation meat products

	Freshwater bass
	Emu
	Cottage cheese (1%)
	Chicken breast, deli
	Chicken breast
Decent Protein Source	Tofu, soft
	Tofu, firm
	Tofu, extra-firm
	Tempeh
	Pork tenderloin, well-trimmed
	Beef tenderloin, well-trimmed
Low-Quality Protein Source	Sausage
	Ground beef (27% fat)
	Bacon

Quality Fats

Your body needs quality fats for fuel to function well. Foods with high concentration of monounsaturated fats, low saturated fats and Omega-6 can provide the best quality of fats. The saturated fats can increase your cholesterol levels that may give way to a heart disease.

Here is a list of good fat sources for your diet:

Class	Food Items
Top Source of Fats	Olives
	Olive oil
	Macadamia nuts
Second Best Quality Source of Fats	Canola oil
	Avocado
	Almonds
	Almond butter
Decent Quality Source of Fats	Peanuts
	Cashews

You can also use butter, lard, safflower oil, or soybean oil only when you have no other choice. It is still best to avoid using any of them as much as possible.

Hold Your Horses!

Before you begin your intermittent fasting, it is best to consult your doctor first and I also recommend that you go to an acclimation period between two and three weeks. This can determine whether intermittent fasting is the answer you have been searching for and help you choose which schedule or type will best work for you. It is a good idea to slowly cut your eating period and not quickly jump to less than 14 hours feeding time.

For the first week, you can set your eating period for 14 hours and then cut it little by little until you only have 12 hours feeding time (recommended for newbies). You can eat anything you want and see how you feel. You can start eliminating unhealthy foods in the next few days and replace them with nutritious fares.

In the next few days, you can try the suggested healthy meal plans below to make your body get accustomed to healthy eating. You have a list of recommended foods to eat. Plan your meal using the list.

For the second week, you may want to try eliminating your breakfast or simply think of it as brunch (breakfast and lunch). You can still have your usual dinner time intact. You may want to cut your feeding time further (aside from eliminating breakfast) or stick to the new schedule.

By week three, you must have your first 8-hour eating window. If it works for you, stick to that schedule. You can also try other type of intermittent fasting if you are not satisfied with the result or savor the experience that you expect to encounter. Just remember that whenever you want to try a different schedule, start slowly to get your body and mind accustomed to your new feeding habit.

Healthy Meal Plans

You can eat normally on non-fast days and it is advisable to have a healthy meal plan. You can plan your meal using any of the following:

1. Follow right portions of quality carbohydrates, protein, fiber, and fat.

You can plan your healthy meal by following the healthy portions of carbohydrates, protein, fiber, and fat. The recommended daily carbohydrate intake is 130 grams or around 43 grams each meal.

The Institute of Medicine recommends about 15 grams of protein per meal for women who weigh around 125 pounds. Men who weigh around 155 pounds should consume 19 grams per meal. Those men and women who weigh more may need to consume more protein. The same goes with those who are physically active.

Adult men who are 50 years old and below should get around 13 grams of fiber per meal, and those over 50 should get around 10 grams each meal. Women who are younger than age 50 should consume around 8 to 9 grams of fiber per meal, and those over 50 should include 7 grams of fiber each meal.

As much as possible, choose quality fats every time you eat to avoid the risk of heart disease. Healthy men and women should include 7 to 12 grams of fat per meal.

2. Plan your meal according to portions by the plate.

You can follow the portions that the plate suggests. You can also use a smaller plate if you want to limit your food. Just make sure that you won't starve yourself while you are still in eating period.

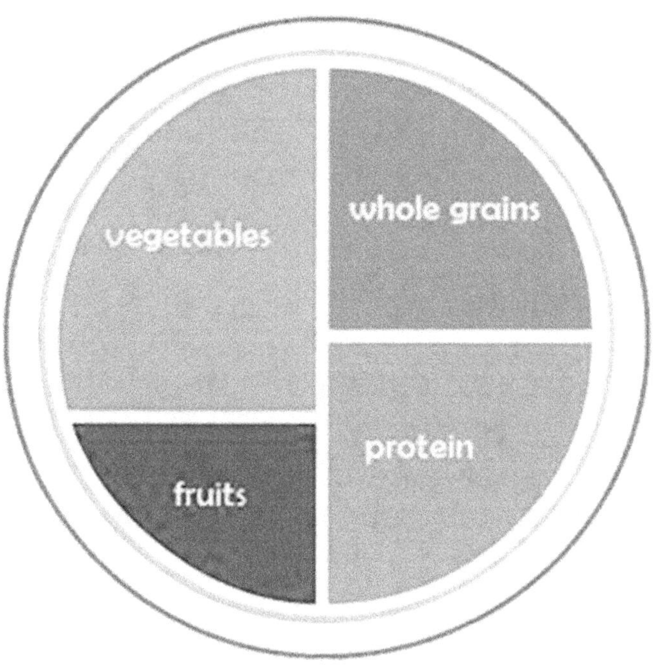

It also helps if you use only plain white plate so you can clearly see the amount of food that you get. When your food has the same color as your plate, you might get more than you need because your brain may experience some trouble distinguishing the right portion size. If you have light-colored foods, it is best to use a plate with dark color.

3. Eat according to color.

If you would like to eat more fruits and vegetables, cover half of your plate with vegetables of different colors and include some fruits. Add some whole grains, healthy fats, and protein on the remaining part of the plate. The colorful combination of different vegetables is appetizing enough to make you want to eat more.

4. Go for salads.

Eating vegetable salads can help you get more nutrients from your diet. You can use the same set of greens with different dressings. You can also use the same dressing for a week for different sets of greens. Although you use the same set of greens or dressing, you will get to savor different taste each time.

You need to create variety to make your salad appetizing and exciting each time you eat it. You can also try experimenting on different vegetable combinations and dressing that go well with each set. You can occasionally add bits of meat to your salad.

You may discover other ways to prepare your meal and make sure to train yourself to eat only nutritious foods all the time. Stay away from sugar, starches, and too much salt.

Foods to Eat on Fast Day

Depending on your chosen method, you may need to modify your meal during a fast day.

It is wise to bulk up on protein to make you feel full for a longer period of time. You can turn to protein as your main source of calories.

You also need to fill your plate with vegetables that are low in calories. They can also help you feel full longer. There are lots of delicious vegetable recipes around and you can always have different dishes every day.

It is advisable to cut your carbohydrates to the minimum during fast day. Carbohydrates may make you feel full but it won't leave you satisfied for a long time. Although fruits are nutritious, it is best to stay away from melon, grapes, bananas, raisins, and other dried fruits during fast days.

You can also include small amounts of quality fats during fast day. Fat can also help you feel full. You need to stay away from fats that won't be able to provide any health benefit.

As much as possible, prepare your own meal so you can be sure about the ingredients that go in it. You need to eliminate chemicals in your daily meals. That's why it is important to buy only organic produce, grass-fed meat, and fresh seafood.

It is also best to consume two to three cups of coffee (best if no sugar and creamer) on fast day. It will speed up your metabolism, cut down your appetite, and make you feel light. Drinking coffee can also provide positive impact on your stamina and strength when you start working out.

Breaking the Fast

It is highly recommended to keep the first two meals of your intermittent fasting meal plan fairly small in size and especially healthy. If you try breaking a fast with a big meal, you will be shutting off fat burning process and making you feel tired all of a sudden.

A big meal during the day won't guarantee that you will be able to keep your hunger at bay. As suggested earlier, it is best to have a protein-rich meal during fast day. You may not have a large meal but you will surely keep hunger under control.

During fast day, your primary aim should be to eat just enough food to keep your body nourished and remain satisfied for a long time without overexerting your digestive system. You will gain enhanced vigor and concentration.

Easy to digest and nutritious foods are good choices to initially break a fast. You can slowly add more variety over time. You can use the list of foods below to help you break a fast. Take note that you may use some in the list within a day or slowly add them within 4 days. You don't need to eat everything in the list, which only serves as the general guideline.

- Vegetable and fruit juices

- Fresh fruits

- Bone broth or vegetable soup

- Cultured milk or yogurt, unsweetened

- Spinach and other leafy vegetables (for salad with light dressing)

- Vegetable soup and other cooked veggies

- Uncooked vegetables (carrot sticks, celery, and others)

- Cooked beans and grains

- Organic eggs and nuts

- Products made from milk

- Grass-fed meats

Pay close attention to your body's reaction to the foods. Stop eating once your hunger has been suppressed. You don't want to feel too full.

When breaking a fast, start with small meals (taken every 2 to 3 hours) slowly progressing toward bigger meals with larger time difference between them. You need to do it until you reach your usual eating routine of 3 meals and 2 snacks in a day.

Remember to chew your food thoroughly. It also helps if you introduce good bacteria (in probiotic) and living enzymes (in fresh, raw foods) into your system.

Chapter 5

Scientific Proof behind Fasting

A body does cleanse itself even without any effort on your part to detoxify it. The best thing about it is that it is a process that you can manipulate. You need to practice a bit of self-cannibalism. You can make your body eat itself via a natural process known as autophagy, which literally means "self-eating".

Autophagy is similar to an innate recycling program within the body. Your cells produce membranes that seek out scraps of worn-out, diseased, or dead cells. The membranes eat the said cells; shred them to pieces to gather usable parts, and use the parts for energy or to generate new parts for the cell.

Autophagy creates more efficient machines to eliminate faulty parts, prevent metabolic dysfunction (like diabetes and obesity), and hinder cancerous tumors. Autophagy is also responsible for decelerating the process of aging.

3 Ways to Boost Autophagy

There are three ways that you can boost your autophagy, and all of them can stress out your body. It may sound weird but stressing your body can boost autophagy. Exercising, fasting, and lowering your carb intake are the best ways to stress your body without creating additional harm.

1. Exercise

When you exercise, your muscles may suffer from microscopic rips that the body needs to heal immediately. Such action makes your muscles stronger and more resilient to any additional damage.

Exercising regularly is the most popular method of unintentionally helping your body cleanse. Whenever you experience a renewed or refreshed feeling after you work out it is because your body has able to cleanse itself via autophagy.

In one **study,** scientists let the mice ran for half an hour on a treadmill and they found out that the mice have increase the rate of demolishing their own cells in a healthy manner. The rate kept increasing until they'd been running for an hour and 20 minutes.

In humans, there is still a need to determine the level of exercise to stimulate autophagy. It is apparent that you can get a lot of advantages when you exercise regularly, aside from ripping benefits from autophagy. It is recommended to perform intense exercise to gain maximum benefits.

2. Fast

Skipping your meal is another way of adding stress to your body (to naturally activate autophagy), in a good way. Research revealed that occasional fast provide many benefits, and some of them may have something to do with autophagy. Fasting can help lower risks of heart disease and diabetes.

There are lots of researches that specifically focus on how fasting effectively promotes autophagy in the brain. The research suggests that autophagy could lower the risk of Alzheimer's and Parkinson's, which are the two most popular neurodegenerative diseases. Intermittent fasting can help the brain improve itself.

Some studies also show that intermittent fasting can improve neuroplasticity, brain structure, and cognitive function. Although it did not explicitly mentioned autophagy as the one that made it all possible, plus the studies were conducted on rodents.

Fasting also triggers stem cell regeneration of old, damaged immune system. The longer you fast, the more benefits you reap. If you think your body is not built for fasting or your doctor forbids it, you can still exercise regularly and lower your carb intake to activate autophagy.

3. Lower your Intake of Carbohydrates

Lowering your carb intake can bring stress to your body and may activate autophagy. Fasting may be difficult for some people, especially those who can but simply won't go as far as skip any of their three meals (plus some snacks).

There is a diet called ketosis that can reduce carbohydrates to a level that compels the body to use fat as fuel. Some say that ketosis is like an autophagy hack.

Properly Digest your Food

There is a need to properly digest your food to avoid feeling tired and sluggish. Your food should only stay in your stomach for about 45 minutes before proceeding to your intestines. You may feel full and bloated when you failed to properly digest your food. You feel tired and lethargic, which should not be the case because food should be able to give you the extra boost of energy and vigor.

Trigger Allergic Reactions

If you don't digest properly, you may develop food allergies or sensitivities. Poor digestion is usually a product of constant consumption of low-quality meats (not grass-fed), too much sugar, and starches. Your body fails to produce needed enzymes for digestion.

Bits of food get handed to your liver. When the liver can no longer manage the overload of undigested food, bacteria, and toxic chemicals, it has no choice but dump the junk into your bloodstream. With all those toxins floating around, your immune system takes action by causing allergic reactions to most substances and foods.

When that happens, the foods that you are allowed to eat become limited and you won't be able to eat as much as you want when you need to.

Chronic Inflammation

Not all inflammation is bad, some swelling happens due to your immune system's response to heal an injury or take care of an intruder. But, when you have poor digestion, this also makes your immune system "on" all the time. It can lead to accelerated aging, swollen joints, and weakened tissue. Over time, it can lead to other ailments including cancer.

It is important to properly digest your food so you won't encounter any problem that may lead to bigger trouble later.

Chapter 6

Gaining Needed Energy and Suppressing Urges

Suppressing urges is the most common problem among people who are fasting. As you grow older, your body becomes accustomed to not giving importance to certain cues. Let me explain further by referring to **an experiment**, which involves children between ages three and five.

The children were separated into age three group and age five group. Both groups were given hefty portions of macaroni for them to eat. The group of three-year-olds immediately stopped eating when their hunger was satisfied. Most of them still have a decent amount of macaroni left on their respective plate. The group of five-year-olds continued eating even if they were already full.

Barbara Rolls of Pennsylvania State University stated that between ages three and five, learned behavior can easily prevail over instincts. The younger children who participated in the experiment instinctively stopped eating when they were not hungry anymore. The older group chose to clean their plate and may have even eaten some more when they saw something good even though they were already full.

From that experiment, we learned that our bodies may have been programmed (since age 5) to ignore the cues. It could be the reason why most people fail to recognize cravings from hunger.

When you are hungry, you won't bother to know what type of food you are eating as long as it's edible. When you are craving for something, you won't get satisfied unless you eat that specific food that you have in mind.

Fat Burning and Sugar Craving

You already know that fat burning does not occur while you are in your eating period. Your body only starts burning fat for energy during fasting period. It means you need to eat in order to gain some fats to burn, and you need to stop eating in order to start burning fats.

You crave for sugar if you didn't eat enough calories or ate the wrong food. Providing the right amount of calories to your body can help you keep your sugar cravings at bay. You can train your body to get satisfied with the right amount of calories that you take in and don't try to eat more if you are not hungry.

Eating even if you are not really hungry is a bad habit that you need to change. Sadly, it is also something that may trigger your craving for sugar. Instead of getting satisfied with the right amount of calories, your body is already used to getting more calories than it normally should. This is all thanks to your incessant eating.

When you follow intermittent fasting, you are not required to eat more than you need to just because it's your eating period. You still need to stop eating when you are already full. You are also training your brain and body to get used to it.

My advice is to stay away from starchy foods. A bowl of pasta that contains too much starch and not enough protein and/or fat may turn into a large basin of sugar. Your body can absorb the calories in the pasta almost immediately and you won't get any satisfaction from it – you will end up craving for more sugar. To avoid this, you need to make sure to add the right proportion of protein and some healthy fat.

What you need to do

To avoid craving and eating more than you should, you can try drinking 1 to 2 glasses of water before you eat your meal. It is also best to drink plain water to quench your thirst.

Choose healthy snacks if you need to have one between meals. Fight the urge to eat junk foods because you will only make things worse. Junk food contains mostly calories, which you must keep under control.

It is recommended to eliminate junk foods in your home or anything that may trigger your craving. Try to stock up on healthy treats that you are usually not fond of. This will be able to help you kill your craving or at least you will get a healthy snack in case you can't control it.

Try to follow any of the suggested healthy meal plans to make sure that you are eating something healthy.

Chapter 7

About Working Out and Exercising

Different people work out best under certain situations. There are people who believe that workout should be done after having a proper meal, while there are also others that think it is more beneficial to exercise on an empty stomach.

Like most enthusiasts of intermittent fasting, I believe that exercising on an empty stomach is more beneficial than working out after eating.

Significant Effects of Fasted State

An empty stomach sets off a gush of hormonal changes throughout your body that may encourage fat burning and muscle-building processes. The two significant effects of fasted state are:

1. Enhanced sensitivity to insulin.

Your body releases insulin each time you eat to help you absorb the nutrients from your food. Insulin draws out sugars from your bloodstream and directs them to fat cells, muscles, and liver to be stored for later use. Eating too often and too much can make your body more resistant to the effects of insulin. Eating less frequently can eventually improve the body's sensitivity to insulin.

2. Increase the body's growth hormone (GH).

GH helps the body improve bone quality, burn fat, and generate new muscle tissue. Fasting, together with proper sleep and weight training, can help increase production of GH.

Why Exercising during Fasting Period is Beneficial

When you exercise during fasting period, your body is being compelled to shed fat. The sympathetic nervous system or SNS controls the fat burning processes of your body. Your SNS gets activated via lack of food and with exercise.

The combination of exercising and fasting can maximize the impact of cellular factors that can influence breakdown of glycogen and fat for fuel. In one study, it was revealed that fasting before undergoing an aerobic training can reduce body fat and weight, while consuming food before exercising can only lead to weight loss and nothing more.

You can start exercising before breakfast if you feel like doing it first thing in the morning. You can schedule your exercise according to your fasting period. Whenever you fast, you may choose to exercise. If you prefer daily intermittent fasting, you can exercise every other day or a couple of days per week – your exercise schedule depends on your fasting period and your preference. The important thing to remember is to keep a regular schedule for your work out to reap the maximum effects.

Eating a full meal, particularly taking in carbohydrates, before you exercise will only inhibit your SNS and diminish the effects of your work out in burning fat. Also, in **another study** those who fasted before they work out had increased levels of a muscle protein that contributes something to insulin sensitivity.

Protein Drinks and Supplementation

There are different protein drinks and supplementation that you might want to try to get the most out of your work outs. Here are some of them:

Egg Protein

Egg protein contributes more than just protein. It is rich in minerals and vitamins that your body needs to function well.

The downside is that there are people who have allergies to eggs and it is one of the most expensive protein supplements around.

Whey Protein

It is known to promote fat loss and lean muscle growth. It also supports healthy metabolism and cardiovascular health. Your body can quickly absorb whey to help you with post work-out recovery.

The only downside to this is that some people may find it indigestible due to the presence of lactose, which some people can't tolerate.

Casein Protein

Casein offers the same benefits as whey, but they have different release process. It takes a longer period of time to digest casein making it the most favorable protein drink before hitting the sack.

Like whey, casein is a milk by-product that contains lactose. Your body absorbs it slowly and it won't perform well during post-work out recovery.

You can also include apple cider vinegar in your diet. It can help you feel more full when you ingest it and make you eat less or suppress your craving.

B vitamins can also help, but make sure to take only the necessary ones. You don't need to take them all.

You may also want to try choline, Conjugated Linoleic Acid (CLA), Gamma-Linolenic Acid (GLA), guarana, green tea extract, L-carnetine, Vitamin D, Vitamin C, Vitamin E, and zinc. Consult your doctor first before you try the supplements just to make sure that you don't have an unknown ailment. The good fats can be found in the suggested list on Chapter 4.

Chapter 8

Sticking to the Course

Now comes another challenge – how to stick to the course. Don't worry, every once in a while most of us feel like we can't go on anymore. Believe me when I say that it's only temporary. You need to remind yourself about the wonderful things that you will gain and don't lose sight of your goals.

I am sure that you already know that you need to focus, choose healthy meals and make your body get used to it, have enough sleep to remain clear-headed, and create variety. It also helps to engage in outdoor activities   and   join   groups   that are interested in intermittent fasting. You can also do the following:

1. Plan your meal carefully in advance and deliver yourself from temptation. Don't let your peers tempt you too.

2. Keep a busy schedule to make time literally fly. Before you know it, another day has passed and you accomplished so much.

3. Keep your body well hydrated to prevent craving or hunger occupy your thoughts.

4. Instead of counting your losses, you need to start counting your victories. You might be surprised just how many times you have overcome obstacles.

5. Don't forget to congratulate yourself for coming out of a successful fast. Other than food, you can treat yourself for a job well done – a vacation perhaps?

You will discover other things to make you stick to the course and always think positive.

Conclusion

Thank you again for downloading this book!

To be blunt, it is not easy to fast and you may only see some results after a couple of weeks. You will gain increased energy level as well as fit and healthy body. It is also possible that you may need to change the type of intermittent fasting that you follow. If you have followed my suggestion regarding acclimation, you should have chosen the most suitable type of intermittent fasting.

To tell you the truth, it took me some time before I was able to find the most suitable type of fasting that I truly prefer. I wrote about acclimation because I went through the process of finding the most suitable one for me the hard way. It came to a point where I almost gave up and I sure am glad that I never did. If I have given up early on, I won't be able to experience all the wonderful benefits that I enjoy today.

I want you to experience the amazing things that changed my life for good. I hope that this book will be able to help you change your life for the better.

If you enjoyed this book, please take time to share your thoughts and post a review on Amazon. It'd be greatly appreciated!

Thank you and good luck!